M000202729

THE PRACTICAL GUIDE
TO THE
BEARD

Other Schiffer Books on Related Subjects:
The Art of the Beard, Angie & David Sacks, ISBN: 978-0-7643-5773-2

Copyright © 2020 by Schiffer Publishing, Ltd.

Originally published as *Le Guide Pratique de la Barbe* by Groupe Eyrolles, Paris © 2016 Groupe Eyrolles
Translated from the French by Simulingua, Inc.

Library of Congress Control Number: 2020930713

All rights reserved. No part of this work may be reproduced or used in any form or by any means—graphic, electronic, or mechanical, including photocopying or information storage and retrieval systems—without written permission from the publisher.

The scanning, uploading, and distribution of this book or any part thereof via the Internet or any other means without the permission of the publisher is illegal and punishable by law. Please purchase only authorized editions and do not participate in or encourage the electronic piracy of copyrighted materials.

"Schiffer," "Schiffer Publishing, Ltd.," and the pen and inkwell logo
are registered trademarks of Schiffer Publishing, Ltd.

Graphic design: Studio Eyrolles
Layout: Hung Ho Thanh

Iconographic credits
Jean Artignan: p. 68 (bottom)
Barbe N Blue: pp. 59, 76, 77, 78, 80, 81, 86
Hung Ho Thanh: pp. 15, 68 (top), 71, 72
Hung Ho Thanh and Jean Artignan: pp. 28, 29, 30, 31, 32, 38,
39, 40, 41, 42, 43, 44, 45, 46, 47, 48, 53, 54 (top), 55, 56, 57, 58
Shutterstock: And-One (p. 74), beboy (p. 25), Cherkas (p. 79), Egudinka (pp. 4, 5, 36, 35 except bottom right), Eugenio Marongiu (pp. 25, 50), glebTv (p. 26), g-stockstudio (pp. 20, 22, 82), Gutzemberg (p. 65), IZO (p. 54 lower left), MatoomMi (p. 37 in bottom right), mimagephotography (p. 33), Nicklay Grigoriev (p. 64), Oleg Gekman (p. 26), Peshkova (p. 27), SFIO CRACHO (pp. 12, 84), Thomas Pajot (p. 52), Viorel Sima (p. 26), wernerimages (p. 34), wideonet (p. 19), Nejron Photo (p. 62), Ander5 (p. 73)
BarbeChic® is a registered trademark.

Type set in Burford/DIN/Archer

ISBN: 978-0-7643-6026-8
Printed in India

Published by Schiffer Publishing, Ltd.
4880 Lower Valley Road
Atglen, PA 19310
Phone: (610) 593-1777; Fax: (610) 593-2002
E-mail: Info@schifferbooks.com
Web: www.schifferbooks.com

For our complete selection of fine books on this and related subjects,
please visit our website at www.schifferbooks.com. You may also write for a free catalog.

Schiffer Publishing's titles are available at special discounts for bulk purchases for sales promotions or premiums. Special editions, including personalized covers, corporate imprints, and excerpts, can be created in large quantities for special needs. For more information, contact the publisher.

We are always looking for people to write books on new and related subjects.
If you have an idea for a book, please contact us at proposals@schifferbooks.com.

JEAN ARTIGNAN

THE PRACTICAL GUIDE
TO THE
BEARD

CHOOSE, TRIM, MAINTAIN

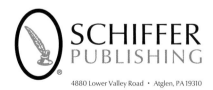
SCHIFFER
PUBLISHING

4880 Lower Valley Road • Atglen, PA 19310

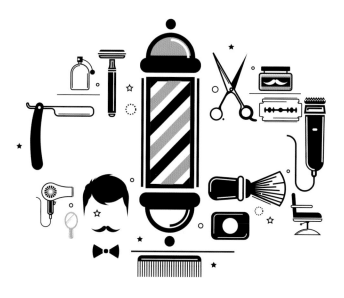

CONTENTS

PREFACE

I'm often asked how to choose a beard style by people who immediately talk to me about the shape of faces, but it's not as simple as that . . .

The diagnosis starts as soon as the client enters the salon. I observe him from head to toe: his style, his walk, his attitude, everything that constitutes his personality. I wonder: What is his job?

Is he a sportsman? If so, what sport does he practice? Alternatively, is he perhaps an artist?

A few questions later, I propose a beard that goes with his identity. It must be part of a whole while adding a peculiarity, since each beard is different, by its growth pattern, its type, and its density; I will therefore need to adjust the size and shape.

Even if his hair is not very well developed, he has several choices, and I explain why: You can opt for a soul patch, sideburns, a goatee . . . this tiny beard can give you a touch of originality and tell a lot about you. If I have an accountant in front of me, he can opt for a rather square beard, round if it is a tender or shy guy, a triangle for a designer—in short, each line corresponds to an identity.

I end up telling him: "You will learn how to trim your beard and play with the lines, whether horizontal, curved, vertical, or diagonal, which will blend with your character traits and the image you want to give, and all that has nothing to do with style or fashion."

For some, a beard will attract the eye away from small details such as a scar or baldness. I've even seen men gain confidence after a stint at the barbershop. I remember one client who was a little reserved but then had grown a beard, which triggered a new reaction. This accessory put him in a dynamic of change and made him want to change his look, especially his clothes or his glasses. Did he feel that people looked at him differently, or was it just the new confidence in him that didn't go unnoticed?

Everything is possible with a beard; the shapes are almost infinite.

We men are lucky in that we can easily test several styles, because a beard is ephemeral. You don't like the shape of your beard? You can just shave it off and start again a few days later without it being a catastrophe.

Today, more and more men are wearing beards and are becoming aware of their possibilities. With this book they will gain in dexterity and will be able to go further by experimenting with more-elaborate styles such as a mustache. Where shaving was considered the morning chore, the maintenance of your beard becomes an intimate moment, a rite in which you take care of yourself. Many products specially designed for beards are also making an appearance, allowing beards to be taken care of and shaped to your liking.

Whether you're looking for the style that suits you best, techniques to trim and maintain your beard, or tips, I hope you'll find in this practical guide concocted by Jean all the advice to accompany you.

I'll finish here with a phrase by Lao Tseu that I like and that guides my beard lines: "There is no better lie than a big truth." In other words, if you have holes in your beard, don't hide them—accept them!

Anthony Galifot

hairdresser–trainer–master barber–ambassador of Barbe N Blues

WHO IS JEAN?

During a holiday period, like many men, I decided to leave my razor at the bottom of the drawer. A few days before officially resuming work, I had to go back to the office to retrieve a document. When I arrived, I met a colleague who said, "Jean? I didn't recognize you; the beard suits you; you should think about keeping it . . ."

So I thought, "Why not?" Even though beards are accepted more and more, in practicing a profession where I was often in contact with customers, my beard had to be impeccable.

At that time there weren't any websites dedicated to beards. Not finding the practical information I needed, I decided to experiment on my own.

After a few botched cuttings and trimmings and many accessories, I discovered some techniques and tricks that I thought would be interesting to share on a blog, and *BarbeChic* was born . . . At the same time, beards started appearing on the faces of actors, sportsmen, and TV presenters.

The number of visits to the site increased rapidly, and the educational articles were widely consulted. It was with a view to highest quality that I began to turn to professionals to gather their experience and techniques. The goal was to enrich the site so that everyone could benefit from the advice of a barber for taking care of his beard at home.

This positioning on a booming profession in France opened the doors of a very small world. That's how I started to participate in various barbershop openings, where I was able to make very nice encounters. I have discovered a world in which good humor is required and where craftsmen talk to me about their craft not as a job, but as a real passion. It was thanks to them that I discovered old-fashioned shaving, and I revived my grandfather's razor to maintain the contours of my beard. I also started testing beard treatments and accessories (oils, shampoos, brushes, etc.).

Then, to meet the growing demand of many visitors, I decided to create an online store where one can find a whole range of specialized products. A few months later, on a beautiful summer afternoon, I received an email: "Hello, I visited your blog. Would you be interested in a book project?" So that's how *The Practical Guide to the Beard* was born. Just like the blog, it offers advice by describing simple techniques to follow step by step to achieve a flawless beard. Nourished by encounters with passionate master barbers, this book contains a bit of each of them.

So whether you are a beginner or an initiate, looking for tips or just curious, I hope this guide will meet your expectations and make you want to experience new things by going even further in personalizing your style and grooming your beard.

Jean

www.barbechic.fr

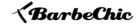

WORDS FROM MEN WITH BEARDS

Before I started this book I wanted to hear the concerns that men have about their beards. It was on a spring afternoon, in the streets of downtown Nantes, that I went to meet them, accompanied by two acolyte beard ambassadors: Anthony (master barber) and Swann (founder of the Barbe N Blues brand). Here is an excerpt of the comments received.

"As soon as my beard gets too long, I can't keep it neat."

"As a guy, I don't know what I want for my hair or my beard. My girlfriend when she goes to the hairdressers', she's able to direct the hairdresser to get what she wants. I wish I could do the same thing with my barber."

"I pay a lot of attention to my beard, but I don't know how to make it look how I want it."

"I have an irregular beard; I would love to wear a beard, but I don't know what style suits me or how to keep it neat."

"I wore the beard, but I shaved since then, because there were lots of drawbacks: over time I get itchy, my beard gets dry, and the hairs get stiff..."

I would love to wear a beard, but it grows white and black..."

"I would like to try a mustache, but I don't know how to shape it..."

As you can see, all men ask questions about their beards. This guide will try to answer your questions step by step to make you a real bearded gentleman!

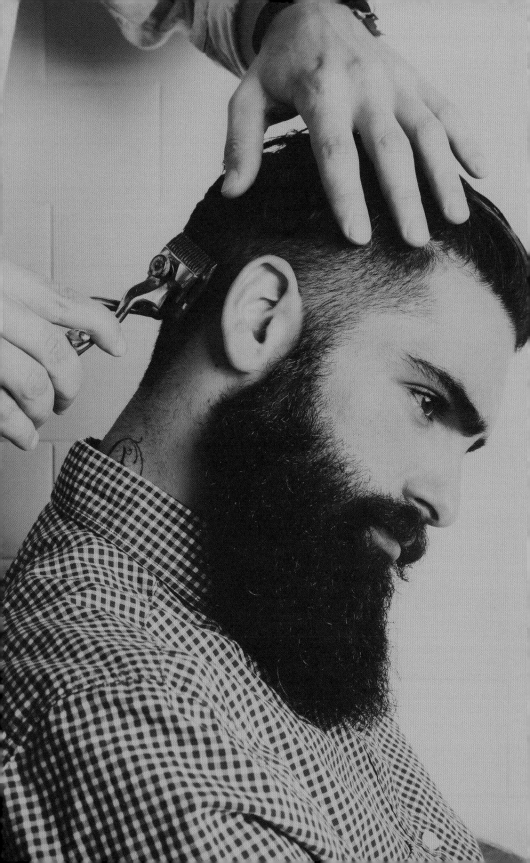

★★★ 1 ★★★
INTRODUCTION

HAIR AND BEARD

In the Beginning . . .

Hair is undeniably a heritage of our ancestors! Like any mammal, they needed thick hair to keep warm.

A few thousand years later, this hair is still present on the entire human body, but hardly visible to the naked eye. Among our five million hairs, the majority take the form of a transparent down, sometimes difficult to distinguish. For example, the forehead is one of the densest areas of the body in hair.

The areas of hair visible on our body consist of thicker and darker hairs, the growth of which is influenced mainly by hormones. The different concentrations on the body still seem to have a function today. Thus, hair preserves the head from the cold, eyelashes and eyebrows protect the eyes from sweat and dust, and hair in the ears and nose acts as a filter against impurities. On other parts of the body they prevent friction-related heating and help evaporate perspiration.

What about Beards?

Like with our ancestors, a beard acted as an insulator to protect the face. Then why is it present in men and not in women, you might well ask. In reality, women have as much facial hair as men, but it is so thin and transparent that we hardly see it. It's testosterone—present in very large quantities in men—that promotes the growth of thicker and stronger hair than women's.

In men, it is during puberty that peaks of hormones accelerate the growth of the beard. These peaks also cause the appearance of hair on other areas of the body and voice modification, marking the transition to adulthood.

Generally, a first down appears above the upper lip at about fifteen years old, then on the cheeks and chin at about sixteen to seventeen years old. A full beard, with maximum facial hair, occurs around twenty years old, or even twenty-five years old, but it can vary greatly from one individual to another.

Hair Structure

The part of a hair about 4 mm below the skin is commonly called a root or follicle, and at its base there is a dermal papilla composed of many vessels. The visible part forms the stem.

The root is in contact with one or more sebaceous glands. These secrete sebum that lubricates both hair and skin to prevent drying. This seborrhea also participates in the formation of the hydrolipidic film, whose main function is to form a protective barrier against bacteria while maintaining skin flexibility.

Beard hairs have the same structure as other hair, but they are thicker on the face than on the top of the skull. They're even the densest of the whole body.

Hair Growth

The life cycle of a hair is broken into three phases. The first phase, youth (anagen phase), is the one during which the hair grows. It starts with the root formation and lasts a few months for body hair, about a year for beard hair, and up to six years for other hair. This is the longest phase of the hair's life cycle. The second stage, old age (catagen phase), lasts approximately three weeks and is transient. The hair is resting, growth stops, and the root slowly begins to disintegrate. The last stage is the death of the hair (telogen phase). This is caused by new hair growth that causes the older hair to fall out. This phase varies according to the body area and individuals. For hair it is estimated to be three months, compared to two months for the beard.

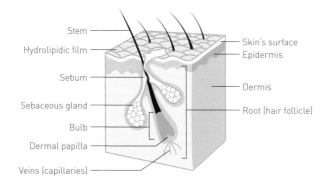

Stem · Hydrolipidic film · Sebum · Sebaceous gland · Bulb · Dermal papilla · Veins (capillaries) · Skin's surface · Epidermis · Dermis · Root (hair follicle)

Beard Growth

The life cycle of beard hair extends for about fifteen months. Each hair is at a different stage: about two-thirds in the growth phase, one-third at the end of their lives, and only a few at rest.

This sequential growth ensures a constant renewal of your beard, which explains why hair loss is not noticed. This gives you the idea that some beard hairs grow faster than others.

On average, beard hair grows 0.4 mm per day, but as always, it can vary from one individual to another. The main factors influencing beard growth are

★ heredity: there is a good chance that your growth pattern resembles that of your ascendants;

★ hormones: estrogen, testosterone, or thyroid hormones have an influence on the life cycle of hair and its thickness;

★ metabolism: deficiencies in vitamins, amino acids, or even mineral salts can slow growth, cause hair loss, pigmentation loss, or excessively fine hair;

★ external factors: stress, medication, sleep deprivation, and smoking.

Misconceptions

After a shave, the hair grows back faster, thicker, and denser.

False—technically the passage of the razor cuts only the hair on the surface; the bulb remains intact, and it is a hair identical to the one you cut that continues its growth.

The feeling of a harder hair comes from its beveled cut and the fact that a short hair seems more rigid, but it will soften as it grows.

If you want it to grow as fast as possible, there is only one solution: let the hair grow without intervening. Some barbers will tell you to trim your beard after a month to reactivate growth.

The use of some cosmetics and pills can increase pilosity.

False—you will find on the market different products that promise you a dense beard. In fact, the influence of these products is very limited. At best, some dietary supplements will allow you to have a slightly silkier, resistant beard that grows a little faster, but it will not grow in areas where it was not previously present. Otherwise a manufacturer would have already made a fortune with a product against baldness! Since the main factors of hair growth and distribution are genetic and hormonal, you cannot do much about the amount or lack of hair.

The only thing you can influence is your metabolism. For this, adopt as healthy a lifestyle as possible, which any good doctor will tell you:

⭐ a balanced diet rich in vitamins, amino acids, and mineral salts;

⭐ regular physical activity;

⭐ adequate periods of sleep;

⭐ moments of relaxation to limit stress;

⭐ no tobacco or alcohol.

These tips may seem generic, but only a healthy organism will allow you to have a resistant beard and hair with an optimized growth cycle.

A daily brush can slightly accelerate growth by stimulating the bulb. But be careful not to abuse it. Once a day is enough; otherwise it will cause the opposite effect—hair loss. Brewer's yeast and castor oil are known to boost growth speed, but this will still not fill the holes in the beard.

For areas with no or little hair, I invite you to follow the recommendations in this guide, which will show you what to do about it.

WHY WEAR A BEARD?

Five Good Reasons

We asked average people why they wore or liked beards, and in many cases it was women who answered our questions when we had a couple in front of us. The most frequently cited are these:

⭐ **Reason #1**: "For comfort; it saves me from having to shave every day. And shaving damages my skin a little."

⭐ **Reason #2:** "It makes me look older, and that's good. I look more mature; otherwise I look much too young."

⭐ **Reason #3:** "I love it! It's manly and soft. I make my boyfriend grow a beard for more than 3 days."

⭐ **Reason #4:** "It's a question of how you look. A real style tool; you can cut it in many ways to change your face . . ."

⭐ **Reason #5:** "It's sexy and trendy. I'm registered on dating sites; I see that beards work!"

A Beard: An Asset for Good Health?

Yes! Or at least it can be an interesting asset, and for many reasons. Your beard acts as an insulating layer that protects you from wind and cold; it prevents your skin from drying out. If you also make sure that your face is well hydrated, it will show fewer signs of aging.

The beard also reduces symptoms related to asthma and allergies. Facial hair, especially near the nose, acts as a filter that traps pollen and ambient dust.

Another positive point of a beard: without shaving, or simply shaving a part of your face, you reduce the risk of irritation, even infection. Some sensitive skin may be the victim of ingrown hair, rash, or inflammation of the hair root. To avoid this, refer to our tips in the chapter "Shaving" (see page 63).

Finally, your beard partially protects you from the sun. Australian researchers have shown that at certain times of the day, beards provide relatively effective protection for hair zones. However, that doesn't exempt you from applying a sunscreen . . .

THE RETURN OF BARBERS

A Little History . . .

Antiquity

It is necessary to go back to the time of ancient Egypt to find the first traces of barbers. At that time, beards were reserved for kings and gods. Generally speaking, men shaved their faces and heads completely. Among the clergy the priests practiced complete shaving as a sign of purity.

The pharaoh—half man, half god—was the only one with a thin and fine, braided beard that was actually false and maintained by his personal barber.

The profession of traveling barbers was common, and, according to the literature, they went from street to street in cities from morning until evening, going from one house to another to shave gentlemen.

This Egyptian expertise has been passed down through the centuries, with the barbers of Cairo being renowned for shaving faces with aplomb and dexterity.

A short time later, in Greece, we find rooms reserved for men where barbers took care of beards and long, wavy hair—very fashionable in those days. In addition to doing brushing and cutting, barbers applied lotions, ointments, and beeswax to hair and beards to perfume and shine them.

The profession of barber quickly gained great success, with shops gradually becoming meeting places of Greek high society to talk of philosophy or politics.

It was not until the advent of the Roman Empire that this noble profession was imported from the Greek colonies to western Europe. With the fashion in Rome having returned to hairless faces, the "tonsors," as they were called, dedicated themselves more and more to shaving. To do this they used a "novacula," an instrument in bronze with a curved blade sharpened with stone, and a simple bowl of water.

From the Middle Ages to the Twentieth Century

It was then necessary to wait for the Middle Ages for a change to take place in the profession. At the beginning of the thirteenth century the church issued a decree condemning surgical acts, thus making them a sin of sacrilege. At the time, doctors were mostly members of the clergy; they were therefore forced to stop interventions.

Barbers, skillfully mastering blades, began gradually to practice small procedures and dental extractions that were, despite this conviction, indispensable. Later surgeons, united in a corporation distinctly separated from barbers, denounced them. They then grouped themselves into a fellowship and established a charter that was ratified by King Charles V. It granted them official status and guarantees to practice their profession of barber-surgeon in peace. Several centuries of battles over the prerogatives of barbers, fed by doctors and surgeons, followed.

THE BARBER'S POLE

The barber's sign reflects the heritage of this trade. This pole was inspired by the blue cane that patients had to hold perpendicular to the ground in order to hold their arms tight and to bring out their veins during bleeding procedures.

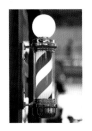

The red color and the spiral evoke the blood-soaked bandages hanging outside the stalls to dry or simply to attract the attention of customers.

In the nineteenth century, it was the bearded dish (an oval dish cut on one side to place it under the clients' chin) or the yellow basin, used for bleeding, that was suspended as a sign.

Today the barber's pole has become the universal symbol of barbers, and you will find it all over the world.

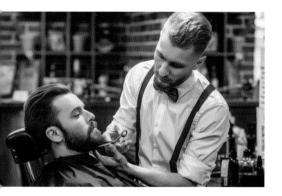

In the 1970s, men wore their hair long, and masculine/feminine salons appeared, leaving little room for real barbershops. Teaching shaving and beard maintenance disappeared from the training programs of apprentice hairdressers.

Today

In the first few years of the twenty-first century, there were generally only a few barbers. Little by little, hairdressers who were passionate about this traditional profession embarked on an adventure, and barber formations reappeared.

It gave rise to multiple edicts and ordinances that gradually reduced the scope of intervention of barbers.

It was not until the middle of the eighteenth century that the kings of France and England made the decision to permanently separate the professions of surgeons and barbers, leaving them only hair care activities.

Although barbers seemed doomed to decline, they experienced a new impetus thanks to the fashion of the wig. These barbers were entrusted with the daily maintenance of wigs, in addition to their manufacture and installation. Worn both by women and men up to the French Revolution, they gave the profession many great years and some recognition.

As a sign of rejection of the old regime, wigs gradually disappeared and barbers refocused on hair care. Then, in the nineteenth century, the profession of hairdresser, whose heirs are the salons we know today, developed.

Nowadays men pay more attention to their look and have become aware that beards can be a real asset to show them off to their best advantage.

This strong return of the beard in recent years (a beard of three days, then a full beard, and more recently the mustache) has given a boost to this trade, and many barbershops have opened. So many that today an experienced barber has become a scarce resource, which could make them very rich in the next few years.

At the same time, beauty salons have launched into the male niche without really breaking through. In fact, health centers and other spas retain a very feminine image among men.

So what's better than a place where you take care of beards—the manly attribute par excellence—to take care of yourself? You don't say, "I just got back from the spa; I took advantage of it to do a facial," but "I just got back from my barber's, who gave me an old-fashioned cutthroat shave."

It should be noted that a barber's ritual certainly gives you a moment of well-being at least as pleasant as in a spa . . .

How to Choose Your Barber

Generally you should prefer salons that claim to employ barbers first, and check the list of services offered. A barber is a barber for men; he mastered the techniques of haircutting, which he learned how to apply to beard trimming during his training. But that's not all: a real master barber practices old-style shaving following the ritual described on page 68.

If you are going to a barbershop, make sure that the person who will take care of you has received barber training, and do not hesitate to ask for his references. Don't go to a salon that has suddenly added shaving and beard care because it is fashionable . . .

There are many styles of barbershop: the old-school type with the rock 'n' roll atmosphere of the 1960s, the traditional type decorated with ancient objects and an old Belmont barber's chair (the reference), the chic and classy atmosphere of the 1920s, New York's industrial design . . .

Some barbers offer facial treatments, a manicure, or other waxing. On the other hand, followers of tradition confine themselves to trimming and shaving. You will also find artisan barbers who trim the beard only with scissors and straight razors, leaving electric trimmers at the bottom of the drawer. It is up to you to choose the one that best suits you, according to your style and expectations.

Your barber is here to show you off in your best light. He should accompany you in the choice of a style of beard that suits you, but he should also give you advice. Don't hesitate to ask him questions.

Don't forget that a visit to the barber should be a moment of pleasure; if you haven't enjoyed the atmosphere or the service, don't hesitate to try other salons to find the one that suits you.

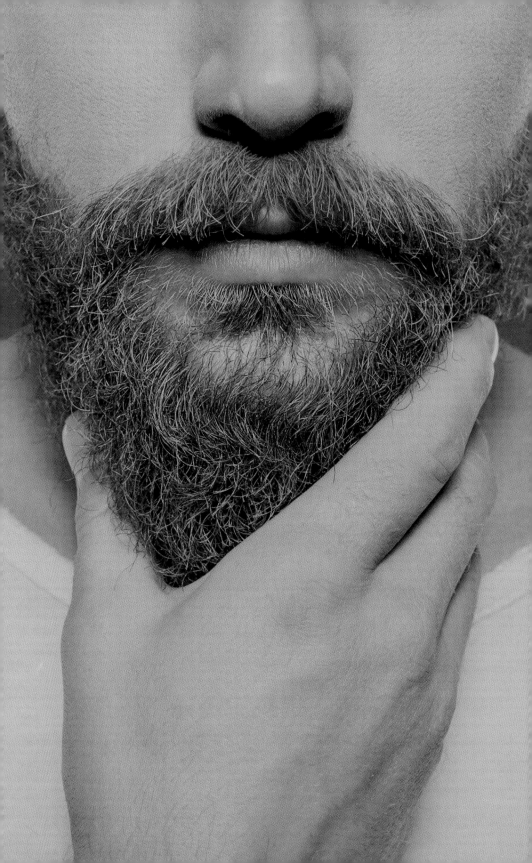

2

CHOOSING YOUR BEARD

TO BEGIN WITH

First of all, know that there are as many beards as faces; growth pattern, type of hair, and color make each beard unique. Let yourself be guided in choosing a beard that suits you.

Overview

First essential step: do a short test. Let your beard grow for a few days and observe your face from all sides. Which areas are dense? Which ones are sparse? In which direction does the hair grow? What about your mustache?

Regardless of what some people say, you have to deal with the material you have and adapt your beard to its growth pattern. Even if it is possible to find products or food supplements on the market that promise an increase of hair, they will be able in the best of cases to strengthen the existing hair but not develop it where there isn't any.

Rather than trying to hide possible holes in your beard, it is better to accept them by playing on the beard line and to draw attention with another detail. Your cheeks are hairless? Why not opt for a goatee, with a stylish mustache and a soul patch. With a beard, anything is possible!

Look and Personality

A beard must be in tune with your identity. Of course it can bring a little extra in the construction of your own style, but it must match your inner self while being in tune with your environment.

The Athlete

Often careful of his style and image, an athlete likes to experiment with assertive looks and change them regularly. Being athletic—V shaped—his choice of beard can often be defined by his body. In this case, use straight lines and angular geometric shapes instead of short beards to avoid the unpleasantness of perspiration: sculpted chinstrap beards and goatees such as judoka Teddy Riner's. But don't necessarily copy all sportsmen: rugby man Sébastien Chabal has adopted a style that makes him look like a caveman . . .

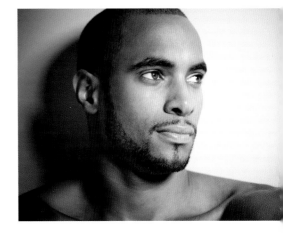

The Artist

Artists have always played with their mustaches, such as Salvador Dalí, who experimented with many styles, or the painter Anthony van Dyck, who, by adding a beard, invented a style of beard that bears his name. Indeed, with the latter there are many possibilities to assert one's personality.

It requires daily care to shape and stylize it, as you can see in the chapter on mustaches on page 51.

To embellish it, why not add a more or less thick soul patch?

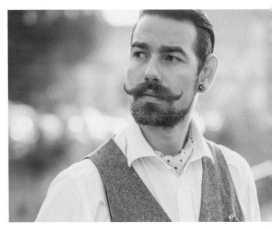

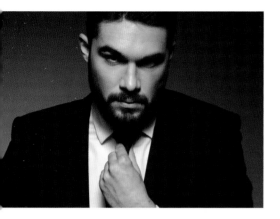

The Young Executive

Whether a man is in a suit with a tie, in an office, or in contact with customers, his having a beard—previously banned—is now accepted, but only on one condition: that it is perfectly maintained. Prefer a full, short beard, taking daily care of the contours so that it stays neat. That doesn't stop you from playing on a few little details that will show your personality, like a sculpted soul patch or demarcation lines that are straight or more curved.

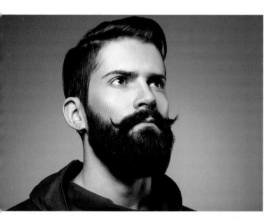

Urban Vintage

Do you collect ancient objects? No doubt you will enjoy the beard styles worn by our grandparents, while giving them a touch of modernity. For example, opt for an imposing handlebar mustache formed with wax and possibly accompanied by a long Nicholas II–style beard.

The Biker

Are you a fan of superb machines and leather jackets? You need a manly beard. Without growing a long beard immediately, you can try a circle beard with sideburns.

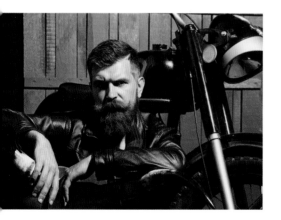

Your Personality

You are unique; the beard styles you will find in this guide are here only to inspire

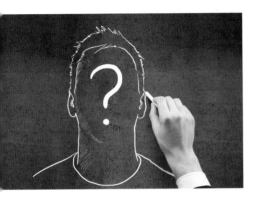

Many books, especially in hairdressing, talk about style of cutting in function of the shape of the face. I voluntarily chose not to discuss this question in detail in this book, because for me, this is not the main criterion for choosing a beard style. As mentioned, the style will depend mainly on your growth pattern, the material you have at your disposal, and your personality.

If you're one of the lucky few who has a kind of beard that offers you all possibilities, just remember some elementary rules and good sense.

The face that is considered the most masculine is rather square, compared to an oval shape for women. If your face is round, for example, play on straight lines to give it angles and avoid beards that are too thick, especially on the cheeks.

On the other hand, if your face is square, do not overuse sharp lines or angles. Choose slightly curved lines that will soften your face. A short beard would suit you perfectly.

If your face is elongated, avoid accentuating this shape with a long beard, a goatee, or even sideburns. Prefer an imposing beard, keeping some volume on the cheeks.

Above all, wear a beard you like and remember that the shape of it also reflects your personality!

you. Your beard must match your personality, so do not hesitate to experiment with several styles and to seek advice from your family and friends or, better still, a master barber. In any case, if it doesn't suit you, you can always shave the whole lot off and try again a few days later.

Beard and Hairstyle

There must be a contrast between your beard and your hair. If you have a sharp beard and haircut, neither your hair nor your beard will stand out.

In fact, if you have an imposing and well-crafted cut, prefer a rather discreet beard, and, on the contrary, if you have a more classical haircut, you can play more with the style of your beard, which will then be the center of attention, making it a true beauty accessory.

PRINCIPAL BEARD STYLES

A Three-Day Beard

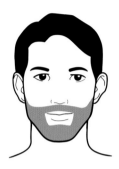

This beard is very successful. Contrary to what one might think, it still requires maintenance to avoid a neglected look. Its length varies between 2 and 5 mm.

Five O'Clock Shadow

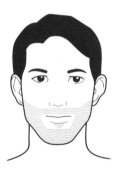

Also called an evening beard or nascent beard, it takes its name from the beard that naturally appears on a shaved face at the end of the day. It is an ultrashort beard of 0.5 to 1 mm. It is better suited to men with dense growth.

Short Ten-Day Beard

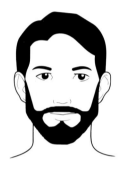

This full beard is suitable for many men. It gives a uniform result that may be suitable for those with low-density growth. This beard can be worn in all circumstances if it is well maintained. It is widespread and therefore less original.

Long Beards

Long beards take several months to grow and can have different shapes according to how you want to look.

Natural

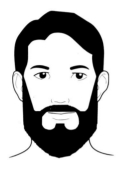

Just let your beard grow according to your growth pattern, remembering to trim the contours to keep it neat.

Ducktail

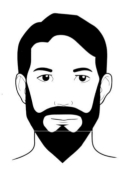

Slightly more sophisticated, this beard is cut in point, at the level of your chin. For an even more distinguished result, you can add an imposing handlebar mustache that will give it a Nicholas II style.

Fork

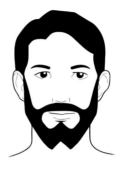

Also called "French fork" because it recalls the two-tooth ancestor of the fork, it is divided into two parts at chin level.

Garibaldi

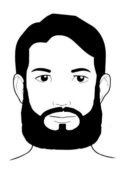

Rounded in shape, this beard can measure up to 8 inches long and gives a more rustic appearance. While the mustache must be well maintained, the growth of the beard on the face is freer.

This beard is maintained with scissors following its curve. Worn without a mustache, with flared sideburns it becomes an Old Dutch.

Sculpted Beard

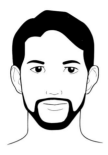

It is a short beard whose contours are perfectly drawn. The mustache, neck, goat, and cheekbones are precisely cut with a razor. It can take many forms, such as a full and short beard, a chinstrap, or a goatee and a mustache. This beard requires daily maintenance and is better suited to men with dense growth.

Goatee

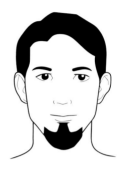

This is a small chin beard that can take different shapes and can be worn with a mustache.

Circle Beard

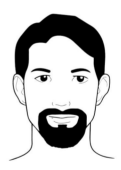

Commonly mistaken for a goatee, a circle beard is a small chin beard that connects around the mouth to a mustache. This style of beard can have several variations by playing on the shape of the mustache to give it a more assertive look.

Hollywoodian

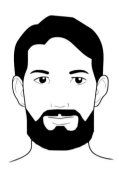

This beard takes on the shape of a short beard, but without sideburns. The demarcation on the cheeks is also lower than on a full beard.

Van Dyck

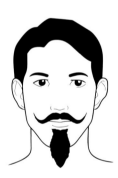

Named after the famous Flemish portrait artist Anthony van Dyck, it consists of a straight beard on the chin and whiskers that are not connected to the corner of the lips. Several variants exist, but the real Van Dyck is a pointed goatee with a well-sculpted and thick soul patch. With longer whiskers and a thinner beard, the Van Dyck becomes an imperial beard or Napoleon III.

Soul Patch

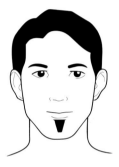

A soul patch is a small beard carved under the lower lip. It can take many forms, such as a triangle, half moon, rectangle … but it often remains discreet. It can be completed by adding a mustache. Lying to form a vertical line in the center of the chin, it becomes a chin strip.

Sideburns

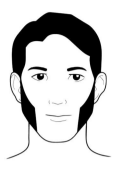

These strips of hair on each side of the face were in fashion during the '60s. Today, they reappear in a more discreet and perfectly sculpted form. They can accompany other beard elements such as a goatee or a mustache.

Anchor

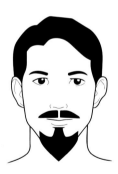

This beard is composed of a mustache, a sculpted chinstrap, and a pointed goatee that can take the shape of an anchor. With a more imposing and rounded goatee, it forms a Balbo.

Captain Jack

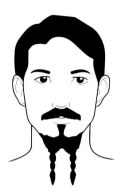

Formed of a mustache and a goatee divided into two braided strands, it is the beard worn by Jack Sparrow in *Pirates of the Caribbean*, the character from whom it takes its name.

Combination

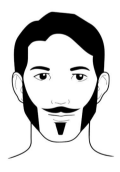

To make your beard unique, do not hesitate to combine these styles, and also pay attention to your mustache.

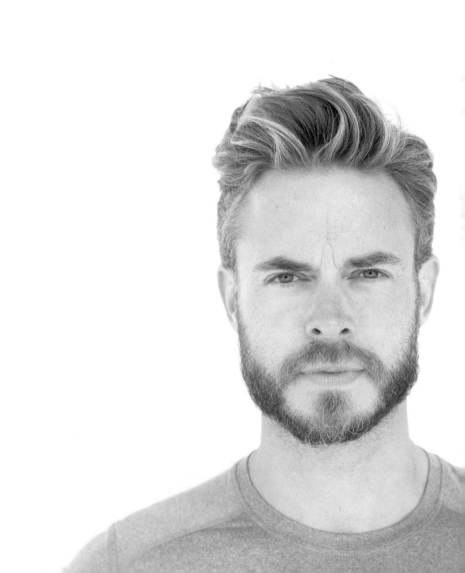

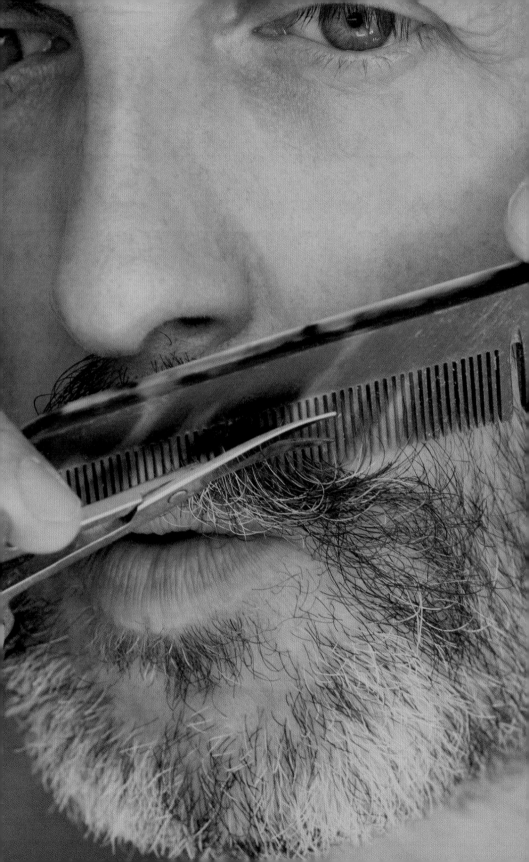

3

TRIMMING
YOUR BEARD

FIRST STEPS

To get started, you have to give your beard time to develop. Since the growth rate of hair varies from one individual to another, it is difficult to tell you exactly how long it will take to grow. On average, one week for a three-day beard, two to three weeks for a medium-sized beard, and two to three months for a long beard.

Since the intermediate stages of hair growth can make a beard look more or less tatty, I advise you to take advantage of a holiday period to avoid any shaving. If presentation is important in your work, you will need to gradually grow the beard by doing minimum maintenance, mainly shaving your neck, cheekbones, and mustache. The goal is to have as much material as possible to shape into the style that suits you.

TOOLS

Clippers

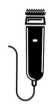

The first indispensable tool, clippers will allow you to sculpt and maintain your beard. To guide you, here are the elements to consider when choosing your clippers.

★ Guide combs and cutting heights: number of cutting heights, interval between each height (0.5 mm, 1 mm, etc.), and type of guide comb (adjustable, interchangeable, without a comb)

★ Load time and autonomy: use this criterion if you are often traveling.

★ Cord or cordless: corded or battery-powered clippers. In the case of cordless clippers, check that it is possible to run them directly connected to an outlet; this is very useful when the battery is completely discharged.

★ Washing method: washable in water for its practical side or with a brush

- Type of blades: stainless steel, titanium/carbon (more durable), or ceramic for increased cutting accuracy
- Accessories and options: transport bag, mini clippers, or precision razor

For starters, I advise you to get cordless clippers with an adjustable comb guide with different cutting heights. This will allow you to explore different beard lengths before finding the one that suits you.

Over time, if you gain in skill, you can acquire professional clippers without a guide, or even with a cord. It will have a longer lifespan than mainstream clippers, but you will also need to learn how to use it to trim your beard with a comb. For the most skillful, scissors can even replace this accessory.

For cordless clippers, count on at least $30 for a high-quality model and up to $80 for the most-advanced versions integrating a razor or suction system.

For professional tools, count on around $30 for a corded model and more than $100 for a cordless model.

Scissors

Essential for neatness, scissors will serve you daily for cutting off rebellious hairs or adjusting your mustache. Scissors specially designed for beards and mustaches are available commercially. In any case, you need small scissors (about 4 cm blades for 10 cm total length), and rather sharp ones to gain precision.

Razor

To maintain the contours of your beard, you can use your usual blade or electric razor.

For more tips on choosing your shaver and the shaving ritual, see page 63.

Comb

Choose a standard double-toothed comb consisting of a detangling part (wide tooth) and smoothing part (fine tooth). It will allow you to comb your beard and will also help you in your alignment.

Avoid plastic combs that generate static electricity, which tends to make hairs bristle. Choose models made of horn, wood, or carbon.

Beard Brush

A beard brush is the essential tool for the bearded, but do not get just any model! Choose a real boar-silk brush.

This type of hair is rigid and antistatic and allows disentangling, smoothing, and tackling beard hair. You get a uniform result. Choose a brush with very dense, short hair bristles for a short beard, and a less dense-bristled brush for a long beard.

TRIMMING TECHNIQUE

To cut a beard is to follow the steps of the ancestral occupation of a stonemason. The latter starts from a block of rough and imposing stone; he observes from all sides to detect its specificities and other irregularities. He thins the whole, having first delimited the contours by means of lines drawn. Then comes the moment of adding the finishing touches, which requires time and dexterity to give the sculpture its final shape.

By analogy with your beard, you should understand that you must first let it grow to have enough material to work.

TRIMMING A SHORT OR MEDIUM BEARD

Contours

For starters, brush your beard well to arrange your hair before cutting. Keep this brush handy, since you will need it between each step to bring out the hair to be trimmed. First, you have to define the contours of your beard. Observe your growth pattern to identify natural boundaries.

To draw the contour, equip yourself with your clippers without a guide comb. When you have finished trimming your beard, you can use your usual razor to get a cleaner result by removing the remaining hairs.

Cheekbones

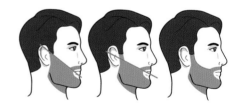

Cheekbone line

Take a comb and place it to draw a line from the top of the ear to the corner of the lips. Use your clippers without a comb guide to remove all the hair above the comb.

To get a cleaner face, you can also go down slightly below this line from the middle of the ear to the corner of the lip.

If the result seems too straight, you can try to cut a slightly curved line that follows your face. Be careful not to exaggerate this rounding; it would bring out your cheekbones and make you look chubby.

Note that since each beard growth pattern is different, the landmarks mentioned above may vary. In all cases, remember this: the demarcation line of the beard must be regular, so make sure to cut it by following your growth pattern, and above all, make sure it is symmetrical.

Neck

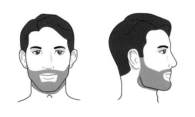

Neckline

To bring out the lines of your face and avoid a neglected look, special attention must be given to the base of the neck. Use your beard clippers without a comb guide to shave a slightly rounded line that follows your face.

To do this, raise your head and start from just below the angle of the jaw on one side to the other side. To do your line correctly at the base of the neck, at the level of the throat consider that your line must be above the Adam's apple at a distance equivalent to the width of a finger (see diagram on the left).

Do not forget to round the angle formed by the beard at both ends of the jaw under the ears (see diagram on the right).

The Beard

Equip yourself with clippers that are adjustable or interchangeable. First use the largest comb guide and then run the clippers over the entire beard in the opposite direction of the growth direction.

Observe the growth direction of your beard; it will surely be necessary to make movements in different directions according to the parts of the face. Generally, the hairs on the cheeks grow toward the middle of the neck, growing downward and slightly sideways, and those from the base of the neck grow upward.

Each growth pattern is different, and you can have horizontal hairs on the jaw, for example.

Continue trimming by successively using a smaller and smaller comb guide or gradually turn the knob of your adjustable guide. Continue until you obtain the desired length—usually 2 to 5 mm for a three-day beard and up to 10 mm for a short beard, ensuring perfect symmetry.

If you find that your beard is not dense enough for a shorter cut, don't insist. To get a neat result, you have to find the length that allows you to get a regular size on the entire face. If you find that some areas are a little denser, you can use a shorter comb guide on these places to thin them and thus balance the whole.

The easiest part is done; now all you have to do is keep your beard neat and clean in all circumstances!

Mustache

It's a matter of style and taste. Some people will prefer to cut it to the same length as their beard, or a little shorter to avoid it being too noticeable. Others will opt for a goatee-mustache style by leaving this area a little denser than the rest of the beard.

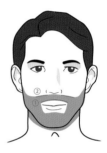

Contours of the mustache

In any case, brush your mustache down with a small comb or a beard brush to bring out the hairs you are going to trim.

Then use small scissors or clippers without a guide to trim the hairs that cover the lips, to obtain a nice contour (1).

If the top of your mustache is a little too thick, especially at the ends, trim it to redesign the contours. Also consider cutting hairs under the nostrils (2).

The use of a shaving soap or foam can mask the contours of your beard. To avoid this, you can use shaving oil. It creates a protective barrier between the skin and the razor blade, but above all it is transparent, so you can visualize the limits of your shaving line.

Caution, because some "preshaving" oils are not used without the complementary application of shaving foam, so make sure to choose oil that can be used alone.

If the area between your beard and mustache (at the corner of your lips) is sparse, you have three possibilities:

⭐ Shave this area shorter so that the link is made by a nascent beard;

⭐ Transform this area by removing this part of the mustache from the rest of the beard. Shave it and make sure not to go too high. Stop at the corner of the lips;

⭐ Accept it! Because trying to hide small flaws often means drawing more attention to them.

Finishing Off

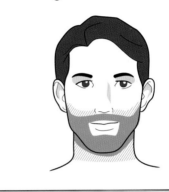

Areas to shave

Shaving

Shave with your usual razor the areas previously delimited at the neck and cheekbones. Do not hesitate to go over them with clippers if necessary. If your skin is too sensitive at the base of your neck and you do not want to shave too closely, then choose an ultrashort cut (0.5 to 1 mm).

Avoid shaving your entire neck under the chin. In fact, the contrast thus created may reveal a double chin that is not very aesthetic.

For an electric shave, the straight-grid models will be more convenient to follow the contours than those with rotary heads. You should also be aware that there are precision grid shavers with a compact head for finishing touches.

Safety razors provide a more accurate and durable shave than electric razors. For an even cleaner result, you can experiment with barber tools such as the straight razor or, for beginners, a shavette (see page 70). In fact, its edge is visible, unlike interchangeable blades, making it possible to see clearly what you are shaving to make precise beard traces.

To reduce the risk of cutting and to shave safely, follow our tips on shaving on page 63

Sideburns

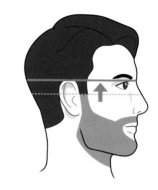

Movement of clippers when trimming sideburns

To get a nice gradation between sideburns and beard, spot the desired level of the sideburns and move the clippers from bottom to top by sliding under the sideburn and going up slightly above the intended limit. You can use markers such as the top of the eyes for the maximum limit of the clippers, and the middle of the ear for the desired height (see diagram).

To avoid accidents, apply the same method as for trimming your beard: start with the largest cutting-comb guide and reduce the size to get the right length. The goal is for your sideburns to blend in with your beard. Do not hesitate to adjust the width of your sideburns to obtain a regular line.

Soul Patch

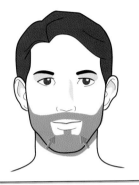

Trimming a soul patch

The soul patch is a small clump of beard under the lower lip. In most cases it is surrounded by small, hairless ovals on each side.

Some hairs grow in the middle of this light zone, and they should be removed for a neat beard. If there are only a few hairs, you can use a tweezers. Otherwise use your clippers without a comb guide or use precision clippers. You have to shorten each side gradually to equalize the whole and get a symmetrical result.

If your chin is completely covered with beard, without any apparent soul patch, you may want to sculpt one. This makes it possible to accentuate facial lines by shaping your chin and bringing out your mouth. Try this if you find that the bottom of your face is too masked by your beard.

Chin and Neck

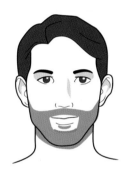

Alternative chin trim

Some men have a beard more or less dense at this spot. If the sides of your chin are denser, cut them a little shorter by adjusting your clippers guide.

JEAN'S ADVICE

To cut the rebellious hairs that protrude from the beard after a few days, you can also use your clippers. For this, use a large guide or adjust the knob to a large size. To avoid straightening the entire beard, I advise you to trim in the direction of the hair growth; for example, from top to bottom on the cheeks. All small hairs that are raised will be thus sectioned. If this is not the case, gradually adjust the cutting size until the first hairs fall.

If the hairs on top of your chin are too sparse, it is sometimes better to trim this area by forming a half moon that follows the shape of the chin, while keeping a small soul patch under the lower lip.

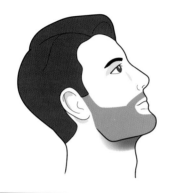

Gradation at the base of the neck

To avoid too much contrast on the lower part of your neck, use the clippers with a guide shorter than your beard length to trim a slight gradation between the shaved area and your beard (see diagram). With a little training, you can prolong this gradation to the entire base of the neck.

To limit the shadow effect below your chin, you can also trim the hairs on your neck a little shorter than the rest of your beard (0.5–1 mm shorter).

Maintenance

Regarding maintenance, it depends on how fast your beard grows. For the neck and cheeks, a daily maintenance is necessary for the beard to remain impeccable. Remember, after brushing, to cut the hairs that protrude from your beard, using scissors. It usually takes four to five days before you need to use your clippers. Always follow the same process:

1 Start by delimiting the "cheek and cheekbone" contours with guide-free clippers.

2 Pass the clippers in the opposite direction of the hair, starting with the largest guide.

3 Gradually reduce the size of the guide to achieve the desired length.

4 Finish with the mustache.

5 Apply beard oil daily to nourish your hair, and remember to shampoo it regularly.

Remember that you can play with guide sizes according to desired density on different parts of the face. Be sure to keep an overall balance, but especially symmetry.

If you're having trouble getting a beard that covers your face evenly, let a longer beard grow or explore other styles!

TRIMMING A LONG BEARD

As mentioned, a long beard requires several months of patience.

The duration of growth will vary from individual to individual, depending on the growth pattern, genetics, and metabolism. While it is growing, follow the contour care tips to keep your beard neat week after week until you get the desired length.

The Shape

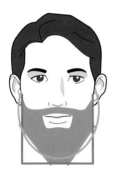

Basic shapes of a long beard

Unless you are a logger's-beard enthusiast, a visit to the barber is almost indispensable the first time. He will give your beard its overall shape, which can be rectangular, curved, pointed, or natural.

Your master barber can also advise you of other styles adapted to your growth pattern that are in tune with your personality.

It is difficult to control an imposing beard from the outset. On the other hand, you will be able to maintain it yourself on a daily basis so that it remains neat. So let's see the essential steps to keep your beard beautiful.

Contours

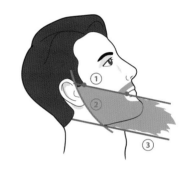

Contours of a long beard

To start, brush your beard in the direction of the hair to untangle it and get any knots out. Then delimit the contours by using clippers without a guide: neck, cheeks (line 1 on the diagram), and mustache, following the same instructions as for the short beard (see the outline step in the short- or medium-beard part).

For a long beard, special attention should be paid to the starting area from the angle of the jaw to the top of the ear. You will need to re-create this natural line with scissors to prevent your beard hair from tickling your ears (line 2 on the diagram).

The most delicate area to maintain

is between the middle of the neck and the chin. It is important to have material in this area, since it supports the beard and ensures a good fit. You still have to maintain it to form a nice beard. To do this, take the lower part of your beard in one hand, lift your head, and cut the rebellious hairs to maintain the line cut by the barber (line 3 on the contour diagram).

The Beard

To make the hairs you need to trim stand out naturally, comb or brush your beard from the root while lifting the hair outward. Then do a few back-brush strokes, especially on the lower part of your face. This way you can easily visualize the hairs standing out from your beard.

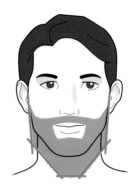

Maintenance trimming a long beard

Using scissors, cut the small hairs protruding from each side of the beard to re-create lines in the extension of the sideburns.

Be sure to keep the scissors parallel to your face. Snipping perpendicular to the face, in the heart of the beard, should be avoided, since doing this would thin your beard and it would lose its uniform appearance.

Style your beard outward again by cutting the hairs that protrude from the rest of the beard. Repeat as many times as necessary.

Use the same method on the lower part to maintain the general shape of the beard. Remember to comb between each snip of the scissors.

Always make a thorough cut and do not use the clippers (except for the contours), because an accident can quickly happen.

If you want a clean result, take care of your cheekbones and neck daily.

If your skin is sensitive, or simply to get a more natural effect, you can test for this area with the clippers without a guide instead of the razor.

Mustache

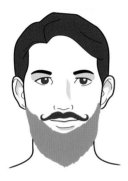

Mustache combined with a beard

Finishing Touches

1. Brush your beard onto your face; use scissors on hairs that are sticking out, keeping the scissors parallel to the beard.

2. Cut the hair that covers the lips.

3. Adjust your soul patch if necessary, so that it is regular and symmetrical.

4. Shave your neck and, if need be, the top of your cheeks.

There are a number of options for the mustache. You can let it blend into the beard or give it a touch of originality by making it stand it out.

For this, let it grow, making sure not to cut the ends, and comb it every day from the center to the outside, on either side of the face.

When you have enough material, use mustache wax to form it. Take a little wax, rub it between your index finger and your thumb to heat it, and then apply it to the mustache from the center toward the outside. Slide your thumb under the mustache at the lips and ends, giving it volume and bringing it out of the beard.

Daily Care

It is essential to renew this global maintenance at least once a week if you want to keep a nice beard. On average a monthly visit to the barber is recommended to re-create the shape of the beard.

Note that a long beard requires more attention than a short beard, so follow our advice in chapter 6 on brushing, shampooing, smoothing, and hydrating it!

SCULPTING A BEARD

You have dense growth, and a full beard bothers you? Do you want to create a style that will affirm your personality more? Let your imagination run free and opt for a sculpted beard. Very graphic, it can take many forms and combinations: goatee, chinstrap, sideburns, mustache . . .

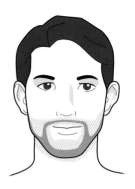

Trimming a sculpted beard

The basics remain the same as for trimming a full beard. Since the contours and lines are particularly visible, it is necessary to take more time and move step by step to create its shape.

For optimal results, start by growing a full beard. Observe your face and visualize the shape of your future beard according to your desires and the growth pattern of your hair.

Create the contours by using the clippers, making sure to leave several inches of margin from the shape you want to get.

Trim gradually, alternating each side of the face, to obtain a symmetrical design. Once you have done the lines, shave the uncovered parts of your face with your usual razor. Use shaving oil for its sliding and transparency properties so you can visualize the limits of your beard.

As sculpted beards are worn short, use clippers regularly to maintain the length of your beard and to adjust its contours.

This style of beard requires a thorough shave and daily maintenance, since small flaws are quickly visible.

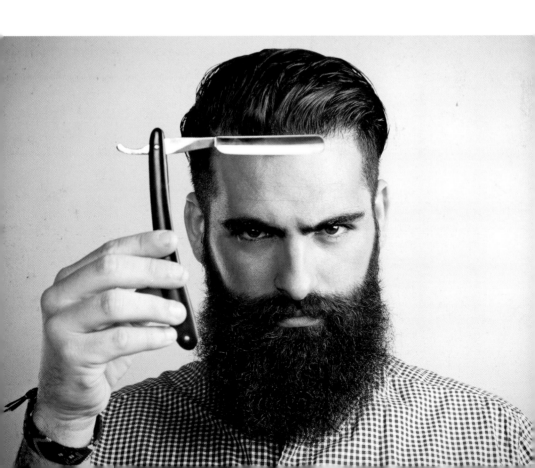

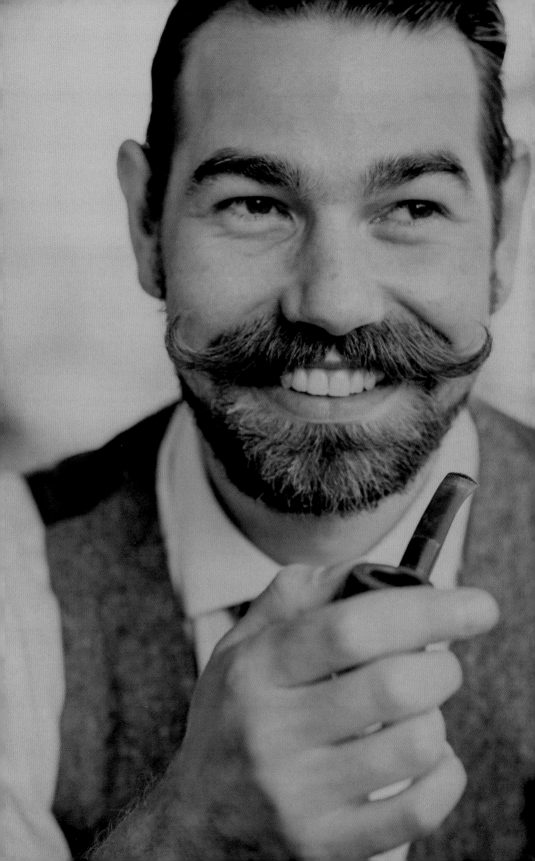

4

THE MUSTACHE

THE MUSTACHE: A SYMBOL

After the success of the beard, the mustache is gradually appearing in the pages of fashion magazines hitherto monopolized by beards. Whether rustic, bushy, or sophisticated, a mustache is a more singular choice than a beard; it attracts the eye and marks the spirits.

Ridiculed for being fuddy-duddy for many years, it has resurfaced in a more elaborate form. A mustache requires a refined maintenance: if it is badly trimmed, it can very quickly make you look scruffy and neglected.

Before you learn how to get a beautiful mustache, study the different styles, keeping in mind that, like the beard, it depends on your natural growth pattern and must be in tune with your personality.

In some countries, almost all men wear a mustache. This is the case in Turkey, where it is seen as a true token of virility and has even become a tourist attraction, since Turkey is a leading destination for mustache grafting.

There is even a popular Turkish saying: "A man without a mustache is like a house without a balcony." Turks also see it as a symbol of political affiliation according to its form: slim, imposing, or stylized. As you can see, growing a mustache can be a serious matter . . .

WHAT IS "MOVEMBER"?

Born in 1999 in Australia, the Movember movement (contraction of Mustache and November) invaded the planet. Have you ever noticed that in November, some men grow mustaches? They are called "Mo-Bros."

Once a year, the Movember Foundation uses the mustache as a means of communication for talking openly about men's health. The multiplication of mustaches on faces in November attracts attention and sparks conversations. It is an opportunity to raise awareness about men's health and to collect donations for

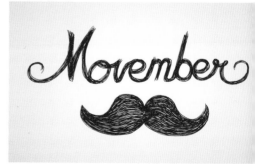

research, but also a friendly and elegant way to do good work. In fact, the media rarely mentions male illnesses, and men tend to consult a specialist once the harm is done.

Movember is aimed at everyone, including women, who can get involved in this male cause. A nickname is even reserved for them: "Mo-Sista." They can communicate with their friends on social networks, collect donations, or participate in the organization of a Movember event in their workplace or at the local university.

The money raised is used to fund programs to prevent and screen for prostate and testicular cancer. Movember is also at the initiative of an international research project, enabling the world's most renowned researchers to pool their expertise to get results faster. This initiative is already bearing fruit and improving the lives of patients by providing them with appropriate treatments.

For more information, visit www.movember.com.

PRINCIPAL MUSTACHE STYLES

Natural

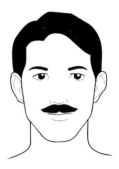

This is the most widely worn mustache in the world and is often the first step toward a more sophisticated mustache.

Natural doesn't mean letting it grow any old way! The idea is to follow your growth pattern while keeping the contours neatly trimmed.

It's up to you to decide how to make it stand out: you can leave it bushy, style it, or add a little wax to make it uniform.

Crustache

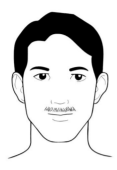

Handlebar Mustache

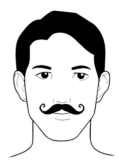

This nickname comes from shortening *crusty* and *mustache*, because it looks falsely neglected. This budding mustache is normally worn by young men who are trying to make themselves look older. This more or less thick down goes with a cool, easygoing look. Keep its length to just above your top lip with a pair of scissors.

This mustache is coming back into fashion. Its peculiarity comes from its two long ends that end curling back on themselves. This mustache is singular and elegant, giving it a little "British" side. When the ends are very slightly raised without forming a curl, it is known as a French mustache.

The handlebar mustache comes in several sizes and can be worn in two whiskers separated in the middle or in one piece. Many men also combine it with a beard. In a fine form with a beautiful three-day beard—or thicker, with a long beard, where it is necessary to give it volume and to form it so that it differs from the beard.

It requires daily and careful maintenance. Some give it its shape by moistening it, but nothing beats a mustache wax to ensure a long, lasting hold.

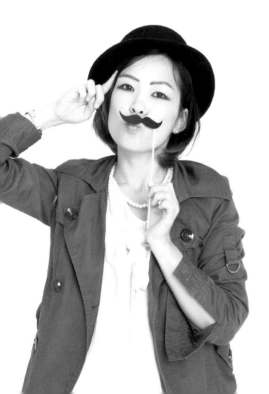

Boot Brush

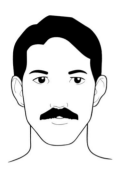

This imposing mustache covers the entire width of the upper part of the lip. Its base is straight and its upper corners are slightly rounded, giving it a shape close to a boot brush.

It is quite simple to maintain; it will be enough to shave daily and maintain its contours with scissors.

Clark Gable

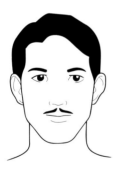

Made famous by actor Clark Gable, this seductive gentleman's mustache is characterized by its fine design, which earned it its nickname "pencil." Several variations exist: the simple line adjoining the upper lip, the curved line perfectly centered between the lips and the nose, or in two distinct parts slightly inclined toward the nostrils.

In any case, it will be necessary to maintain a thickness of a maximum of 3 mm and to trim it with patience and precision to give it its full effect.

The Biker

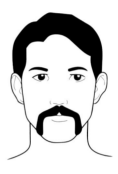

This mustache in the shape of a horseshoe is the attribute of virility par excellence. It may seem a little outdated, but if it is enhanced with sideburns it can dress the face of a man with a shaved head.

Its thickness and width vary according to the desired style: rather dense and imposing for a virile effect, or fine and short cut for a more elegant and discreet effect. For the former style, it is best to start from a full beard or a broad goatee and then gradually give it its characteristic shape.

The Pyramid

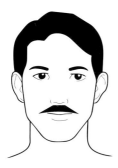

This very geometric mustache is prized by purists. The basic shape is a triangle whose upper part is cut. From this base, several variations are possible, from the small pyramid (whose upper part is narrow and whose two parts meet in the middle of the nostrils) to the more imposing pyramid, the upper part of which will cover the entire width of the nose and whose base will extend beyond the corner of the lips.

This mustache style requires a bit of practice before starting. To shape it, create the top line under the nose and the bottom line above the lips, then form the angles on each side. Finally, shave the contours well to enhance it.

The Fu Manchu

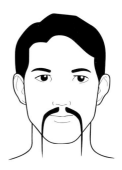

This mustache of Asian origin owes its name to Dr. Fu Manchu, a fictional character (invented in 1912 by Sax Rohmer) who is the villain in many films in the twentieth century. Atypical, it is adopted by some literature students who are fans of martial arts or of Asia.

To obtain it, cut your mustache in two parts, then, day by day, let the ends grow at the corner of the lips. Maintain the contours daily and wait several months. As soon as you start to have a little bit of length, you can use mustache wax to standardize it.

The Chevron

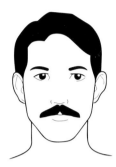

The chevron is an imposing mustache, the upper parts of which are slightly drooping—a bit like the roof of a house—with rounded ends that descend just below the corner of the lips.

This is the mustache worn by Tom Selleck in the *Magnum* series or by the singer of the band Queen, Freddie Mercury.

It is quite easy to achieve but requires concentration while trimming the upper part and rounding the ends.

The Englishman

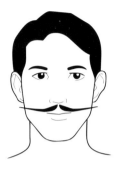

To say the least, this sophisticated mustache doesn't go unnoticed! Thin and elongated in shape, it finishes in well-waxed tips to keep it in shape throughout the day. In a wider and thicker form, it becomes a Hungarian mustache.

To trim it, follow the instructions of the handlebar mustache and apply the wax to form the horizontal tips.

The American

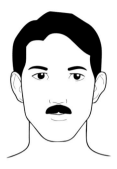

Worn by GIs during World War II, this half-moon mustache still has its followers such as actor Brad Pitt, who regularly wears it even when not filming. To begin, cut the overall shape following the natural curves of your face. Then concentrate on the upper part to form the rounding.

The d'Artagnan

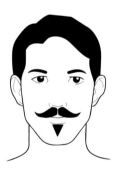

This musketeer's mustache consists of a slightly raised French mustache at the tips and a triangular soul patch. It is more emphasized when you have long hair, especially if you want to try a longer soul patch.

To trim the soul patch, let your beard grow under your lips for a few days. Then proceed step by step, gradually shortening each side until you get the desired geometric shape, then shave the contours.

TRIMMING AND MAINTAINING YOUR MUSTACHE

In this section you will find basic tips for trimming your mustache.

Do not hesitate to complete them with the indications specific to each mustache style and the advice given in the shaving chapter.

The Essential Material for a Neat Mustache

★ **Mustache scissors:** pointed, they are specially designed to thin and sculpt a mustache.

★ **Mustache comb:** compact, with tight teeth, it is ideal to discipline the most recalcitrant hairs and give a uniform appearance to your mustache.

If you use a manual shaver, try shaving oil for its transparency properties. It will allow you to visualize contours during shaving and avoid missing a spot masked by thick foam. If you use clippers, make sure your face is dry before using it.

⭐ **Mustache wax:** This distinguishes novices from enlightened amateurs. It is an indispensable product when you adopt a style that requires a particular shape like the handlebar mustache.

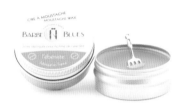

⭐ **Electric clippers:** Not mandatory, but these can be easier to use than scissors when you are a beginner. It is also more practical to draw a very fine or straight outline and to thin your mustache.

⭐ **Razor:** Several possibilities are available to you, such as the interchangeable blade shaver, the safety razor, and the straight or an electric razor. If you are a beginner, use your usual razor. I advise you to turn to bladed razors that are more precise to maintain contours.

First Steps

One of the easiest ways to get a beautiful mustache is to start by growing a full beard for a couple weeks. This will make it easier for you to trim the whole.

To begin, observe the growth pattern of your mustache. For your first mustache I advise you to opt for the natural, so you can see after a few weeks of growth if you have enough material to wear a more sophisticated mustache.

1 Visualize on your face the shape of your future mustache. If necessary, draw this shape with your finger to visualize it better.

2 Use the clippers without a guide or your usual razor to clear your cheeks and neck, making sure to keep a margin of several centimeters with your final mustache shape.

3 Continue to shave, gradually approaching the desired shape. As soon as you are close to it, dry your face if necessary and move on to the next step.

Trimming Techniques

If you have chosen a fine mustache such as the Clark Gable or a very graphic one such as the pyramid, use clippers without a guide to shape the contours. In other cases, if you are skilled enough, you can try scissors. The elements to be taken into account according to the desired style are

★ the upper part of the mustache, following the natural growth pattern, rounded or sloping contours;

★ the lower part, just above the lips, trimming the hairs that grow over the lips;

★ the width, more or less flared horizontally;

★ vertically, more or less downward at the corners of the lips: 1 mm above for most styles, 1 mm below for the chevron and the Fu Manchu, and several centimeters toward the chin for the biker.

Continue with successive small movements on both sides of your face to equalize the whole. Regularly comb your mustache after a few scissor snips to see the hairs you need to trim.

Now that your mustache has been shaped, all you have to do is style it.

Styling Your Mustache

To shape your carefully trimmed gentleman's attribute, nothing beats mustache wax.

Composed mainly of beeswax, it nourishes, protects, and fixes your work of art.

1 Start by dampening your mustache and giving it its general shape with a brush or comb.

2 Take a little wax and rub it between the thumb and index finger of each hand in small circles to heat the wax and make it more malleable.

3 Apply it to the mustache from the center to the ends.

For example, if you want to get a handlebar mustache, use your thumb and index finger to form the tips, as if you were tightening a screw. Then bend them in on themselves to form a loop.

Maintenance

A mustache requires careful maintenance to look good.

★ To do this, back-comb your mustache to lift it and trim anything that protrudes from the comb.

★ If you want to thin it more, comb deeper into the mustache. You should know that for it to be bushy, it takes an average of one month of growth.

★ Comb your mustache in the direction of its growth pattern and trim the contours with scissors. Renew as many times as necessary, remembering to trim the hairs that grow over your lips.

★ If you want to keep your mouth visible, you can trim a 1 mm edge between your upper lip and mustache, along the entire length or just at the ends.

★ To give your mustache the best setting, shave the rest of your face.

A gentleman with a mustache should carry out this maintenance every day!

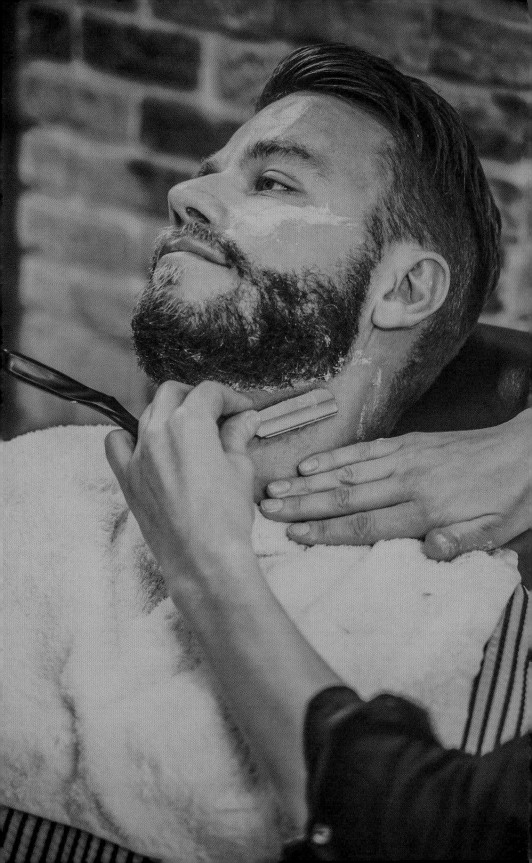

★★★5★★★

SHAVING

A chapter devoted to shaving in a book about beards may seem surprising at first, but for a beard or mustache to look good on your face, your contours and neck area must be well maintained. Here are some tips on how to get an accurate shave while respecting your skin.

TYPES OF RAZORS

Shaving has been practiced for millennia. In the past, razors were made of flint, bronze, or iron. Today there are four most commonly used razors: the electric razor, the interchangeable-blade razor, the safety razor, and the straight razor.

Electric Razor

If you choose shaving with an electric razor, you have the choice between a rotary head razor or a vibrating-blade razor. It all depends on the nature of your beard hair and how much time you want to spend shaving . . .

The rotary head razor was invented by Philips in 1939. It is made up of round heads with rotary blades. This type of shaver is particularly suitable for soft beards; it ensures a quick and accurate shave, even for a week's-old beard. If you have sensitive skin, some redness may appear, usually on the neck.

The vibrating razor has a rectangular head equipped with a microperforated foil under which blades oscillate. When the hair enters the holes, it is cut by a ramp of small blades. This is the system adopted by Braun and Panasonic shavers.

This razor is particularly suitable for hard beards. Shaving takes a little longer than with a rotary head shaver, but some people also find less skin irritation.

Mechanical Razor

The interchangeable-blade razor is one of the most widely used today; there are heads ranging from two to several blades. Manufacturers compete with each other to improve them from one year to the next.

The average lifespan of a blade is five to seven shaves. This depends on the type of hair, since men who have a hard beard will have to change blades more often. Generally, as soon as you feel that your blade is snagging or not cutting properly, it's good for the trash.

Since blades are disposable, they must be purchased regularly. There is also a completely disposable model where the handle is inseparable from the blade. There are also two other types of razors that are making a big comeback among traditional shavers: the safety razor and the straight razor.

The safety razor is the first mechanical razor to appear on the market. It was invented in the early twentieth century by the American King Camp Gillette. It works with very thin blades that are disposable—a great novelty at the time—and it is still marketed today by the brand of the same name. It was very successful because it was in direct competition with the straight razor, which required regular sharpening, and cutting one's skin was more frequent.

The **straight razor** has several nicknames: cutthroat, open razor, or saber. It is the traditional tool par excellence.

Terribly accurate, sharpening it and handling it safely takes time and practice.

TRADITION VERSUS MODERNITY?

Each type of shaving has its fans, so let's see the pros and cons of each, as well as the reasons why men adopt them.

Electric shaving was invented nearly a century ago and has since won a lot of followers. It is done on dry skin, without prior use of foam or other shaving soap. It doesn't cut your skin and rarely causes redness (this does not prevent you from following the ritual of aftershave to take good care of your skin).

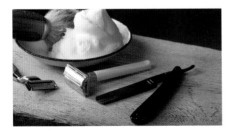

A lot of men find it faster to use, even if the end result is less precise than its traditional counterpart.

Manual shaving, also known as mechanical shaving, is considered one of the most accurate and effective methods. It is carried out on moist skin; the water softens the hair and the skin, facilitating the passage of the blade. It therefore offers a clean and lasting result. This direct contact of the blade with the whole skin is not without its drawbacks. The main adverse effects encountered are cuts, redness, and the appearance of small pimples or ingrown hairs. Note that after several weeks of shaving of this type, the skin naturally gets used to it and discomfort lessens.

THE BEST WAY TO LIMIT ADVERSE EFFECTS

Even if some skins are more sensitive than others, there are some simple steps to follow to limit the appearance of these small inconveniences. Just follow the guide.

When Should You Shave?

It is advisable to shave in the morning, and especially before breakfast. In fact, the blood influx caused by chewing can increase the risk of irritation.

For a manual shave, shave after your shower to soften the hair and epidermis first.

An electric shave is done before the shower, on a very dry face. The hard hair will have more chance to enter the grill and be cut at the first pass of the razor. For this, you can apply a slightly moistened alumstone on the face; its astringent effect will dry the skin and make the hairs stand up.

How to Avoid Cuts and Irritated Skin

As mentioned, shaving after showering is an excellent way to reduce the number of blade passages and the risk of redness.

If your beard is too long, first pass the clippers without the guide on the areas to be shaved, so the number of passages will be limited.

Apply shaving oil, forming a protective barrier between the hydrolipidic film of the skin and the razor while ensuring an optimal glide.

The alumstone is ideal for reducing redness and stopping bleeding. You can also get it in the form of sticks, called hemostatic pencils. Although most of the time the cuts are superficial, the bleeding can still be impressive.

First, rinse your face with very cold water; this will tighten the pores of the skin and blood vessels. Then dry with a paper handkerchief to avoid water accelerating the bleeding.

Moisten the alumstone very lightly and apply it to the wound by using small circular movements; you will feel a slight tingling.

The alumstone has antiseptic but also astringent properties, which stop bleeding and limit infections.

In addition, use soap or shaving cream in a bowl.

Last tip: try to shave in the direction of the hair as much as possible, to prevent the razor from snagging hairs.

How to Avoid Ingrown Hairs

An ingrown hair is a hair that grows under the epidermis, without breaking through it. It manifests itself by the appearance of a small spot that can become infected. To avoid it, here are our tips:

★ At least once a week, scrub your face. Specially designed facial-scrub products, also known as "scrubs," "exfoliants," or "disinfectants," are available on the market. They will allow you to clean the pores of your skin, making it less thick and therefore less prone to imperfections, including those of your beard.

★ Hydrate your skin regularly by applying face creams that are adapted to your skin type.

★ Shave in the direction of your growth pattern.

★ Avoid pressing your razor too hard, and prefer two-blade razors over five-blade razors. In fact, the appearance of ingrown hair often results from a hair cut too short.

★ Follow our shaving tips and regularly change your blade to keep it sharp.

The blade's passage

Hair shaved too closely to the skin

Hair growing under the skin

Ingrown hair causing a spot on the skin

The formation of an ingrown hair

THE OLD ART OF SHAVING

The return to tradition, the desire for a precise shave, and trying to save money are all reasons that lead to experimenting with the shave practiced by master barbers.

You may have discovered, when tidying up your grandfather's belongings, a strange sharp and foldable object—it is a straight razor. In addition to offering an ultraprecise shave and real baby skin, it is very economical. Many fans have found that the purchase of a straight razor is profitable in less than a year, compared to the regular purchase of blades in supermarkets.

Let's take a look at the equipment needed to do this shaving at home, while keeping in mind that it remains an ideal tool to accurately shape the contours of your beard.

The Material

Straight Razor

The authentic straight razor is a unique object that transcends time and can be passed down to future generations. This ancestral tool, still widely used throughout the world, has its own vocabulary, as you can see from this diagram.

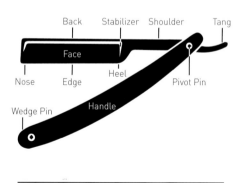

Nomenclature of a straight razor

Beyond the nomenclature, the blade of the straight razor alone possesses many characteristics.

The nose: The tip of the blade can take many forms: rather round (French nose), square (straight nose), or slightly cut (Spanish nose). The rounded shape formed by a French nose allows you to go over the entire face by limiting the risk of injury, and this is the preferred model for beginners. The square-tipped ones allow you to shave areas that are more difficult to access or to make more-precise contours, but their right angle is also sharper.

The face of the blade is also important because it plays on the weight. If you are a beginner, choose a semihollow blade that will be a good compromise between maneuverability and inertia of sliding on the skin. The size, expressed in $^1/_8$-inch increments (1 inch = 2.54 cm), indicates the width of the blade and also has an influence on the weight. The $^5/_8$ is the most common and is ideal for beginners. A narrower blade, such as the $^4/_8$ blade, will be useful for beard contours or to trim a mustache, but it also accumulates foam faster, resulting in more frequent rinsing.

HOW DO YOU GET A SHARP BLADE?

A real straight razor should always be sharp enough to shave and slide on the skin without snagging hairs. Some commercially purchased shavers are labeled "Shave Ready," so they can be used immediately. Those that do not bear any such mention require preparation before use. In any case, your razor will require maintenance before each shave.

You should differentiate between whetting or sharpening, which consists of putting your razor on different grain stones to re-create or maintain the razor's edge (to be used once a year) or whetting on a special leather that will favor sharp edges and thus re-create a regular bevel on both sides of the blade.

For the first use, arm yourself with patience and start by sharpening your razor with the help of leather: 150 passes on the rough side of the leather (on which you will have previously distributed a thin layer of abrasive paste for straight razors) and 150 passes on the smooth side of the leather, without abrasive paste. On a daily basis make thirty to forty passes to maintain the edge of your blade. If you need more details, such as sharpening and polishing equipment and movements, please visit my shaving page at www.barbechic.fr/rasage/ or ask for advice from fans of the Coupe Chou Club forum: www.coupechouclub.com.

Steel: there are two types of steel:

⭐ Stainless steel is hard and difficult to sharpen but remains sharp for a long time.

⭐ Carbon steel is softer and easier to sharpen but needs regular maintenance to remain sharp.

You should count on spending $100 to $150 for a good model.

Shavette

In a country of true old-fashioned shaving fans, the interchangeable-blade shavette is often decried. It is considered to be less efficient and far removed from the traditional timeless object whose edge is sharpened by the hand of man, but it remains a quick and economical way of getting started. For a very reasonable starting budget (between $10 and $35), it allows you to acquire the movement of traditional shaving by considerably reducing the risk of cuts (the blade only exceeds 0.5 mm).

This razor, which is shaped like a straight razor, works with interchangeable blades (safety razor blade cut in two), thus saving you the bother of sharpening it like a traditional razor.

Shavettes are popular with barbers because they allow a precise shave while guaranteeing impeccable hygiene. The blade is changed in front of the customer to show that a new one is being used.

Shaving Brush

This small brush with a very bushy head is essential to prepare your skin before shaving. It makes very creamy foam and distributes it evenly on your face while lifting the hairs before shaving.

The best models are those made from real badger hair. In fact, the natural hair soaks up water and creates beautiful foam. If you are against using animal products, there are high-performance synthetic-hair models.

To optimize the lifespan of your brush, do not hesitate to invest a few dollars in a support. Stored upside down, the brush will dry naturally, avoiding mold and limestone buildup.

Beard Soap

In its shaving bowl, beard soap is the best product for a gentle shave. Its foam lifts the hair and ensures an optimal glide during the passage of the blade. You can also use shaving cream, which foams easily, forming a thick layer on your skin. However, shaving cream doesn't last as long as shaving soap.

Alumstone

Known for many years for its astringent virtues, the natural alumstone calms razor burn and stops the bleeding of small cuts. For small lesions, you can also use a hemostatic pencil.

Preparation

The preparation is at least as important as shaving itself. Follow the following recommendations, which will explain how to shave in peace and obtain a (almost) perfect result.

1 Clean your face to remove impurities and sebum. You can also use a scrub. Shaving efficiency will be better.

2 Dip your brush in warm water and moisten your face to dilate pores and soften hair.

3 Use your brush to moisten your beard soap. Do circular movements with your brush to create nice, thick foam.

4 Generously apply the foam to the areas to be shaved, making rectilinear movements against the hair. This will soak the root and soften the hair.

5 Beforehand you can apply shaving oil to make the blade slide easily.

Shaving

Before you get your razor, keep in mind that it is a sharp object and must be handled with care! Here are some recommendations to avoid accidents.

★ Make sure your environment is calm. Shaving is a relaxing moment that requires concentration. For example, avoid having to watch your children during this ritual, and avoid doing it at the last moment, when you tend to be late in the morning . . .

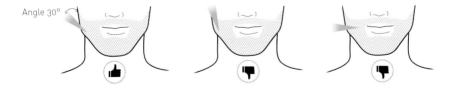

Angle 30°

Angle of the blade

★ Never make sudden movements. If the razor is caught by a hair or nick, do not insist on continuing, and remove it slowly.

★ Keep in mind that a moving blade is less dangerous than an immobile blade. If you don't have a reason to stop, make a slow and continuous slide. When you stop, you are more likely to cut yourself.

★ Do not press or slide the blade lengthwise like a knife; you risk cutting yourself deeply.

★ Before you embark on this ancestral shaving, do not hesitate to consult a master barber so that he can show you how to proceed.

Finally, the long-awaited shaving moment! Before wetting your skin, take note of the direction of the growth of your hair and spot the densest areas.

❶ Grasp your razor, with handle pointing upward, ring finger on the tang, index finger and middle finger on the shoulder, and the blade perpendicular.

❷ Pay attention to the angle that the blade forms with your face. For an optimal result it must be 30°. Pressed against your skin, the blade may not cut the hair; applied perpendicularly, you can nick yourself.

❸ Start your shave with your cheeks, in the direction of the hair—that is to say, slightly oblique, from the top of the face to the neck. It is important to stretch the skin of the face: on the one hand, to remove the folds that could lead to nicks, and on the other hand, to make the hairs stand out.

❹ Proceed in the same way on your neck, always with the skin tight, in the direction of the hairs' growth, usually from bottom to top, and thus from the base of the neck to the middle. Then up and down, from your chin to the middle of your neck.

❺ For your chin and mustache, shave sideways, from left to right if you are right-handed and vice versa if you are left-handed.

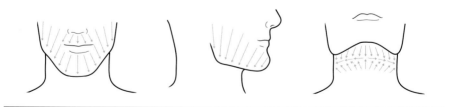

Direction of the hairs' growth

Continue like this for the other shaving parts. Be sensitive to strategic areas such as the corner of the lips, dimples, mustache, chin, and Adam's apple.

If you need to go over your face again, rinse your face first, apply more shaving cream, and shave against the hairs' growth.

Aftershave

The passage of the blade on the face cuts the hair but also damages the surface layer of the epidermis.

The hydrolipidic film that protects the skin from drying out and bacteria getting in is damaged; irritations and other microcuts may appear.

In this case, rinse your face with cold water or apply a cool, wet towel. If there are small cuts, bleeding, or severe redness, apply a lightly moistened alumstone.

Then apply an alcohol-free aftershave balm, having previously reopened the pores of your skin. For this, apply hot water or a small towel soaked in warm water to your face.

Some people use talc instead of or as a supplement to aftershave balm to dry and soften the skin, but it can also clog pores.

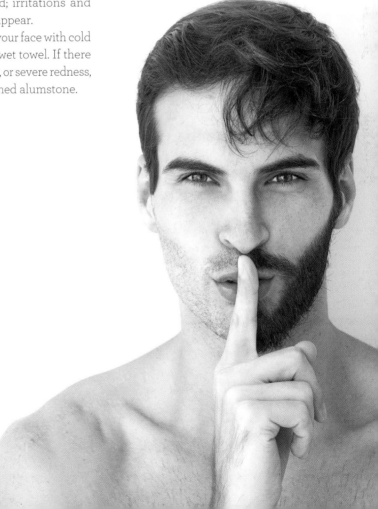

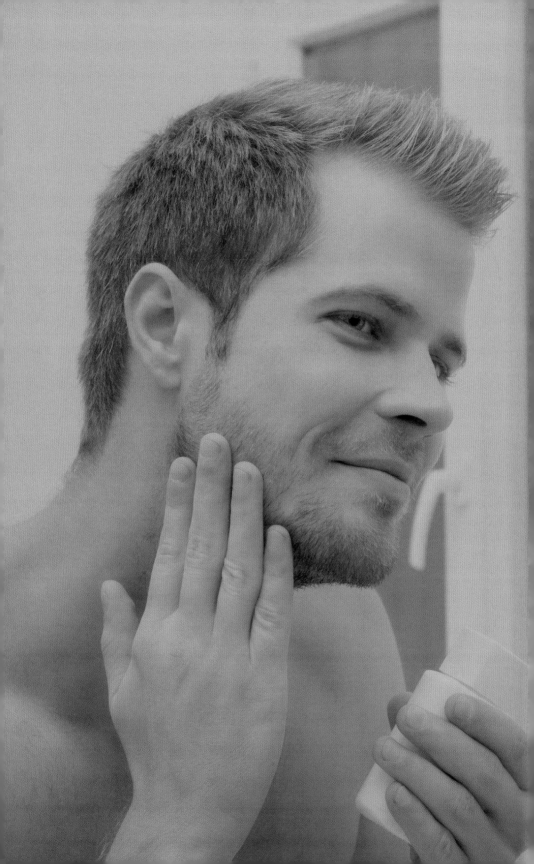

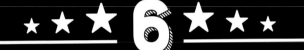

TAKING CARE
OF YOUR BEARD
AND SKIN

Beard hair is delicate; the maintenance of its balance requires several daily rituals that will give it resistance, shine, and flexibility. Like hair, the beard needs to be washed, brushed, and hydrated.

Having a nice beard is fine, but if you don't take care of what's around it, all your efforts will go unnoticed. The skin of your face is fragile and requires special attention.

Let's take a look at the five steps needed to take good care of your beard and skin.

SHAMPOOING YOUR BEARD

Throughout the day, your beard accumulates bacteria. The small gestures of everyday life, such as kissing, eating, smoking cigarettes, or passing your hand over your face, deposit impurities. It is therefore important to clean it to keep it healthy and silky.

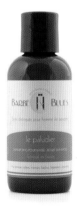

Choice of Shampoo

First of all, be sure to select the right shampoo. Most widely available shampoos contain washing agents (detergents), foaming agents, preservatives, and additives. This combination of chemical ingredients is intended to remove excess sebum from the scalp.

This formula is far too abrasive for your beard and the skin of your face, which are more fragile, and are not even good for frequent use on head hair.

The selected treatment must be soft enough to respect your face and eye contour. Choose a special beard shampoo made of natural ingredients.

Some are even labeled organic, but make sure to take a good look at the composition to ensure the absence of synthetic products. Don't forget that your beard is under your nose, so remember to select a fragrance that you like.

You can also opt for soaps usable both on your face and on your beard. In any case, carefully check the composition of the products and avoid those containing sulfates, silicones, and paraben.

If you use a shampoo based on natural ingredients, it may not foam much, which is due to the fact that it does not contain foaming agents (which also tend to sting the eyes). However, that doesn't stop it from cleaning your face and beard, and the result is plain to see.

Washing

1. Moisten your beard and face with warm water.
2. Apply your shampoo to the entire beard.
3. Massage by making circular movements and making sure to also reach the skin on your face under your beard.
4. Leave on for a few minutes and rinse with warm water.
5. If your beard tends to curl or if your skin or hair is oily, try to wash yourself with colder water. Generally avoid hot water, which would attack the skin and weaken your beard hair.
6. Dry your face and beard thoroughly by tapping it with a towel, or possibly with a hairdryer kept at a good distance.
7. Repeat the operation on average three times a week.

CLEANING YOUR FACE

It is generally advisable to wash your face morning and evening. Cleaning removes impurities such as sebum and pollution from the skin. You can possibly use a special beard-and-face soap if you want to kill two birds with one stone.

In addition, it is important to do a face scrub at least once a week.

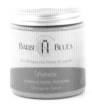 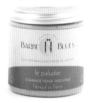

What Is a Face Scrub?

A face scrub comes in the form of a cleansing gel composed of small abrasive grains that act by rubbing to smooth the skin. Often neglected by men, this weekly care has real advantages:

★ It thoroughly cleans the skin by eliminating impurities.

★ Applied to a beard, it gets rid of dead skin that accumulates under the hair—a possible cause of itching.

★ On shaved areas, it stops the formation of ingrown hair and spots.

To do this, use "exfoliating" gels. Make sure they are marked "special face," because body scrubs are far too abrasive.

BRUSHING YOUR BEARD

To obtain a uniform beard, you need to comb it every day.

Note that hair is very sensitive to static electricity, so it can stand out easily. To avoid a bushy beard, it is better to equip yourself with the right accessory. So forget about synthetic combs and opt for real horn combs, or better yet, a natural-hair beard brush.

The best ones are those made from wild-boar hair, because they have very rigid hairs that have several advantages:

★ They untangle, smooth, and tackle the beard for a neat result.

★ They remove dead skin and thus revitalize the skin, which is cleared of impurities.

★ The action of brushing on the skin will stimulate sebaceous production to prevent your skin from getting dry.

Also note that regularly brushing your beard accelerates its growth, stimulating the hair at its roots.

Daily Care

❶ Always brush a dry beard, because brushing a wet beard can break the hair.

❷ Always comb in the direction of the hair growth, on as large a surface as possible.

❸ Massage more or less firmly depending on the desired effect on your skin.

❹ Keep a small beard comb with you to keep your beard neat during the day.

SMOOTHING YOUR BEARD

To smooth your beard, one of the most efficient techniques consists of brushing it the same way you do your hair.

1 Wash your beard with a beard shampoo, then rinse it with cold water, which closes the scales of the hair and thus offers protection.

2 Avoid blow-drying a dry beard, since it will weaken the hairs. It should be damp; dry it coarsely by tapping it with a towel. An alternative exists: you can first apply beard oil to a dry beard before smoothing it.

3 Use a wild-boar hairbrush, if possible round.

4 Use a hairdryer set to the lowest temperature level.

5 Start brushing your beard in the direction of the hair growth by placing the hairdryer perpendicular to the brush and well away from the hair.

Be careful not to get too close to your face, or you will burn your beard and your own skin!

6 Pull the brush down while continuing to dry, and then reverse the movement to dry the underside of your beard.

7 Repeat this movement two to three times per zone.

8 Finish by applying beard oil to moisturize your hair after using the hairdryer.

To avoid damaging your beard, do not overbrush it—limit yourself to once a week.

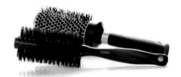

JEAN'S ADVICE

A beard balm, which has a denser texture than oil, will even out your beard better while nourishing it.

NOURISHING YOUR BEARD

Beard hair is delicate; maintaining its balance requires a supply of nutrients to give it resistance, softness, and suppleness.

For this, you can use beard oils that are composed of essential oils and vegetable oils with nourishing, protective, and softening properties. There are high-quality beard oils on the market that have a delicate scent.

You can buy beard balm that in addition to the nourishing effect will discipline rebellious hairs, making your beard uniform and easy to comb.

❶ Place a few drops of oil or a small amount of balm in the palm of your hand.

❷ Briefly rub your hands together to spread the product and heat it slightly.

❸ Apply to the entire beard by massaging it with circular movements.

❹ Make sure that with your fingers, you reach the skin masked by the beard.

If desired, apply the oil or balm to your neck to soothe skin that has razor burn. Nourish your beard daily for optimal results.

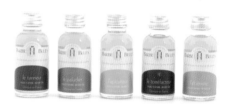

JEAN'S ADVICE

Use an oil or balm, preferably after trimming your beard, shampooing, or showering. In fact, the heat of the shower will have opened the scales of the hair, which will hydrate in depth. You can also use a brush to spread the oil over the entire beard.

HYDRATING YOUR SKIN

Many men tend to forget to take care of their skin. Shaving, using clippers, the cold, and the sun are all factors that weaken the epidermis and can cause redness and dryness.

Exposure to hard water often results in tight skin. To remedy this, you have to nourish your skin daily, preferably at a time when it is clean and slightly damp, after showering or shaving. The skin pores are dilated for maximum hydration.

If you have a short beard—a three-day beard type—you can use a balm or moisturizer for your entire face. Be sure to massage your face well to make the cream penetrate and avoid residue on your beard.

If you have a full beard, opt for beard oil, taking care to make sure it penetrates the skin concealed by the hair. You can use a cream for the parts of your face that are not covered in hair: forehead, cheeks, nose, and especially the neck, the latter being particularly sensitive and weakened by shaving.

If you have sensitive skin, choose moisturizers or aftershaves in the form of cream or balm, avoiding gels or lotions (which often contain alcohol). Alcohol is used in many masculine products for its antiseptic properties, freshness, and astringent properties. It is therefore inherently drying and irritating and can cause tingling, dermatitis, and redness.

If you're sensitive to chemical compounds, there are many natural products on the market. They are composed of in-

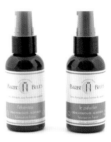

gredients such as oils or vegetable fats, known for a long time for their soothing, antiseptic, nourishing, and restorative properties. The most-common raw materials are shea butter, beeswax, or aloe vera.

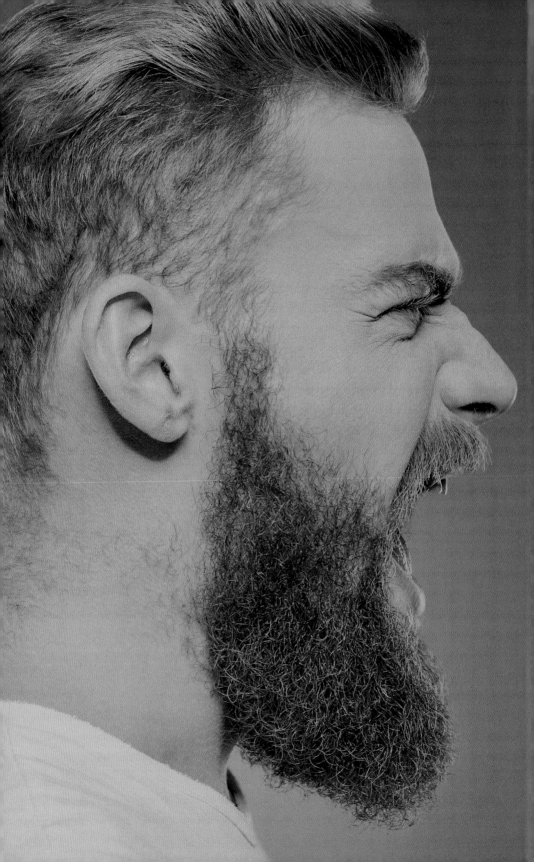

★ ★ ★ 7 ★ ★ ★

HELP!

It is great to have a nice, well-kept beard. Unfortunately, it can sometimes cause some inconvenience. Don't panic; in this chapter we will try to find an answer for your main concerns.

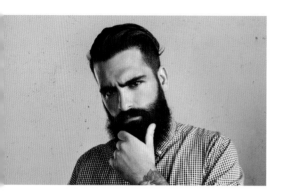

MY BEARD ITCHES

Many men who grow beards complain of itching. The causes can be multiple; let's see some frequent cases and how to solve them.

Are you just starting to grow your beard? Know that it is normal to feel some itching. In fact, first beard hairs are rather stiff and begin to bend and rub against your skin, creating tingling. Generally it takes a few days for this feeling to disappear.

Do you already have a full beard? Be sure to clean your face of dead skin with a brush, wash it, and especially moisturize it (see chapter 6, "Taking Care of Your Beard and Skin," page 75).

Does the itching persist despite following these tips? You may be using one or more products that are not adapted to your skin type. Do not hesitate to change your care to find the one that will best suit your skin, choosing soft and alcohol-free products.

If, in spite of this, you notice itching or redness, do not hesitate to consult a dermatologist.

MY BEARD IS STIFF

There are as many types of beard as hair. Some people have more or less thick hair, and it is the same for a beard.

Have you just started growing your beard? This is normal, because although each beard is different, there is a constant: a short, three-day beard is always more rigid. Try to let it grow a little more so that it will soften.

Do you already have a longer beard? Be sure to brush it regularly and moisturize it with beard oil. Consider using beard balm more particularly adapted to rebellious hairs; it will even out your beard thanks to its thick texture, while also moisturizing it.

MY BEARD IS IRREGULAR AND SPARSE

We are not all equal when it comes to hair. Hormones and heredity have an influence on the distribution of our hair. If your beard is sparse or irregular in places, there are several possibilities.

Do you have the right trimming technique? Use a shorter trimming technique to compensate for the lack of hair and thin, denser areas.

Are you sure of your choice of beard? If your beard is sparse or irregular, you must adapt. Grow more around the sparse area and comb it to make it uniform. Play with beard styles to find your natural growth pattern. Test several lengths and styles, without hesitating to ask your friends for their opinion. You can also ask a barber for advice.

In summary, the best advice we can give you is to accept your beardless areas. By trying to hide a defect, you could eventually make it more visible. On the other hand, you can attract attention to some details of your beard or a nice mustache and draw the eye away from a few imperfections.

MY BEARD IS DRY

Is your beard dry like straw? It definitely needs to be hydrated. To start, try to reduce the frequency of shampooing, which removes the sebum necessary for the natural hydration of your hair. If you use a hairdryer regularly, keep it at a safe distance and lower the temperature.

In all cases, apply oil or beard balm daily. Refer to chapter 6, "Taking Care of Your Beard and Skin," page 75.

Are you on vacation? It is often in the summer, with the trio of sun, sea, and pool, that changes appear. Prolonged exposure to the sun will damage your beard hair by making it dry and discoloring it. Chlorine and salt present in water will dry out and weaken your hair by stripping the sebum that covers it. It is therefore essential to protect your beard from these elements to avoid ruining your care efforts.

Here are some tips and tricks that will be very useful to you. To protect you from UV rays, a simple solution is to apply your usual oil or sunscreen spray to the hair zones. I also advise you to wear a hat and avoid prolonged sun exposure between noon and 4 p.m., which has harmful effects on your skin.

Sunblock

A cool hat

Beard shampoo

Beard balm or oil

A little beard brush

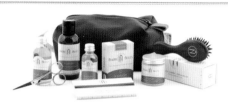

For reducing the effect of chlorine and salt, if you can't resist keeping your head above water, follow these tips. First of all, before swimming,

⭐ apply sunscreen oil; it will form a protective barrier around your beard;

⭐ or soak your beard with clear water; for example, by taking a shower. The hair thus saturated with water will absorb less chlorine or salt.

After swimming,

⭐ rinse your beard, hair, and face for several minutes;

⭐ at the end of the day, shampoo and nourish your beard with oil;

⭐ to finish, brush it to be impeccable for your nights out!

MY BEARD HAS A TENDENCY TO TURN REDDISH OR WHITE

Do you have a red beard? Many men— for example, those having naturally brown hair—have found copper hairs in their beards, caught in the act of turning reddish. Let us try to understand what it really means.

The scenario is often the same: your beard grows, and as soon as it reaches a certain length, red reflections appear. The latter are, at first, visible in the light of the sun, then with time the copper color emerges more, particularly in your sideburns.

I can already hear you saying, "But I'm not a redhead." That's true; well, not quite—you're certainly half red. To understand this phenomenon, researchers have immersed themselves in our DNA, especially a gene in chromosome 16. If this gene is present twice, then you are a redhead; if it is present only once, then you are likely to see red hair growing on your body; and if you do not possess this gene, you're unlikely to have copper hair.

Because genetics do not explain everything, it should be noted that the color of your beard can be influenced by other factors, such as sun exposure and self-tanning creams.

Is your beard white? As with hair, white hair can appear in the beard at any age, and it is not unusual for the first to appear around thirty years of age. Even if they make us realize that youth is not eternal, this process is quite natural and will concern you eventually.

It seems that some factors such as stress, inheritance, and iron deficiency may be responsible for the early onset of white hair.

Although it is easy to remove them when there are only a few, don't forget that it will be more and more difficult to hide them over time.

What are the solutions? There are, as with hair, dyes to color your beard. You will then have to identify the color that will give you a natural appearance. Above all, think about maintaining the roots, because, as you will have noticed, beards grow fast.

Avoid hair color products; since beard hair is thicker and drier, it will be harder to color. Since the beard is less dense than the head hair, hair products can also color your skin. Opt for specially designed beard colors that will look better on beard hair and will respect your skin.

And if you just accept it? You can decide to accept the color of your beard and be proud of it, since it adds to your singularity and will save you a lot of hassle in maintenance. In addition, if it makes you feel any better, many people are fans of the "salt and pepper" look.

I BOTCHED TRIMMING MY BEARD

Anyone can make a false move with clippers or a razor, resulting in an irregular beard. A beautiful beard is a highly symmetrical beard, so you have to make up for your mistake by playing on shape or length. To accomplish this, do the following:

★ Try to equalize the shape of your beard, alternating the longer and shorter parts by adapting the comb guide on your clippers;

★ Take advantage of your mistake by trying another style;

★ Play with the lines of your beard; for example, turn a botched straight line into a slightly curved one;

★ As a last resort, opt for an ultrashort beard or shave the whole lot off and start again in a few days.

WARNING

All the techniques described in this guide are designed to advise you on trimming, maintenance, and shaving your beard.

The tools that are presented, especially those intended for shaving, should be handled with caution and kept away from children.

Neither the author nor the publisher or its partners can be liable for any damage caused by misuse.

In any case, do not hesitate to consult a professional who will initiate you in the techniques described in this book.

ACKNOWLEDGMENTS

I could not have finished this guide without thanking the many people who supported me throughout this adventure and made this project possible:

Anthony Galifot for his wise advice, but also for having relaunched barber training in France a few years ago; Swann Balan, founder of Barbe N Blues, a magnificent range of natural beard treatments; Barbers Abder Blackbeard, Damien Bournique, Rudy Dars, Alex Haircut's, Fatih alias Ottoman Barber, Sébastien Paucod, and Clara and Greg for sharing their passion with me; Frédéric de Planète Rasoir, organizer of the straight-razor day and certainly the most passionate of us all; Gilles de Thiers-Issard for reviving my grandfather's straight razor; and Aude and Jeanne of Eyrolles Editions for having taken on a very masculine subject.

I would also like to thank my loved ones for their many reviews and comments: Amélie, Fred, Marie-Aude, Stéphane, Christophe, Sébastien, Nadège, Charlotte, Rémy, and Guillaume; my parents, who support me in all the projects that I undertake; my wife, for having supported me during writing and hearing all about beards from morning to night; and a nod to Olivier and Matthew for our past and future projects.

Finally, a big thank-you to the readers of *BarbeChic*, without whom this project would not have been possible.